DRUG ADDICTION RECOVERY GUIDE

Healing from drug addiction

Steve Davis

All right reserved
No part of this publication may be reproduced,
distributed or transmitted in any form or by any
means including photocopying, recording or other
electronic or mechanical method without the prior
written permission of the publisher, except in the
case of brief quotations embodied in critical
reviews and certain other non commercial uses
permitted by copyright law
Copyright © 2023 by Steve Davis

Table of Content

Introduction

Drug addiction is a complex problem that affects not only the individual, but also their loved ones and society as a whole. It is a chronic condition that often requires long-term treatment and support. The good news is that recovery from drug addiction is possible with the right approach and resources. This book will provide a comprehensive guide on healing from drug addiction, including understanding addiction, seeking treatment, and maintaining recovery.

Drug addiction, also known as substance use disorder, is a chronic and complex condition characterized by compulsive drug seeking and use, despite the harmful consequences. Addiction to drugs can have devastating effects on an individual's physical, mental, and emotional health, as well as their social and occupational functioning.

Drug addiction is not limited to illegal drugs, but can also include the misuse of prescription drugs or over-the-counter medications. Commonly abused drugs include opioids, such as heroin and prescription painkillers, stimulants like cocaine and methamphetamine, and depressants such as alcohol and sedatives.

The factors that contribute to drug addiction are multifaceted, including biological, environmental, and psychological factors. Individuals who have a genetic predisposition to addiction, have experienced trauma or stress, or have a history of mental illness may be more susceptible to developing a substance use disorder.

The signs and symptoms of drug addiction can vary depending on the type of drug being used, the frequency and amount of use, and the individual's unique physiology. Some common signs of drug addiction include:

- A strong desire to use drugs
- Using drugs even when it causes problems in relationships or at work
- Tolerance, or the need to use more of the drug to achieve the same effect
- Withdrawal symptoms when not using the drug
- Spending a lot of time obtaining and using drugs

Drug addiction can be a serious and chronic condition, but it is treatable with the right interventions. Treatment may involve a combination of medication-assisted therapy, behavioral therapies, and support from peers and loved ones. It's important for individuals struggling with addiction to seek help from a medical professional or addiction specialist to develop an individualized treatment plan that addresses their unique needs and circumstances.

Drug addiction, also known as substance use disorder, is a condition in which an individual becomes dependent on a substance to the extent that they experience intense cravings, compulsively seek out and use the substance, and continue to use it despite negative consequences.

Drug addiction is a chronic and relapsing condition that affects the brain and behavior, leading to changes in an individual's mood, thoughts, and physical health. The use of drugs can lead to a wide range of negative consequences, including but not limited to impaired judgment, financial difficulties, relationship problems, legal issues, and physical and mental health problems.

Drug addiction can affect anyone, regardless of age, gender, socioeconomic status, or ethnicity. It is a complex condition that is influenced by a range of factors, including genetic predisposition, environmental factors, and psychological factors.

Effective treatment for drug addiction typically involves a comprehensive, individualized approach that may include a combination of medication-assisted therapy, behavioral therapies, support groups, and other supportive services. It's important for individuals struggling with addiction to seek help from a medical professional or addiction specialist to develop an individualized treatment plan that addresses their unique needs and circumstances.

Chapter 1

Understanding Drug Addiction

Chapter 1 of this book will provide an in-depth understanding of drug addiction, including its causes, effects, and the factors that contribute to its development. Addiction is a complex and chronic condition that affects individuals from all walks of life, and it is important to understand the underlying mechanisms and processes involved in order to effectively address it. We will explore the different types of drugs and their effects on the body and mind, the cycle of addiction and how it impacts the brain, and the role of genetics, environment, and personal factors in addiction. By the end of this chapter, you will have a comprehensive understanding of addiction and its complexities, which will serve as a foundation for the rest of the book as we delve into the process of healing and recovery.

What is addiction and how does it develop?

Addiction is a chronic and progressive brain disorder characterized by compulsive drug seeking and use despite the negative consequences. It is a complex issue that arises from a combination of genetic, environmental, and personal factors.

In the early stages of drug use, individuals often experience a sense of pleasure or euphoria. This is because drugs can activate the brain's reward system, flooding it with dopamine and other neurotransmitters. Over time, however, drug use can alter the brain's chemistry and structure, leading to changes in behavior and decision-making.

In particular, addiction affects the prefrontal cortex, the part of the brain responsible for decision-making, self-control, and impulse regulation. With repeated drug use, the prefrontal cortex becomes less active, while the brain's limbic system, which is responsible for emotions and motivation, becomes overactive. This creates a powerful drive to seek and use drugs, even in the face of negative consequences.

The development of addiction is influenced by a range of factors, including genetics, environment, and personal history. Studies have shown that individuals with a family history of addiction are more likely to develop the condition themselves. Other risk factors include early exposure to drugs, social and peer pressure, stress, and trauma.

In addition, individual characteristics such as impulsivity, sensation-seeking, and low self-esteem can increase the likelihood of developing addiction. While the exact cause of addiction is still not fully understood, it is clear that it is a complex and multifaceted issue that requires a comprehensive approach to treatment and prevention.

Types of drugs and their effects on the body and mind

Drug addiction is a complex and multifaceted problem that affects millions of people around the world. Different types of drugs can have a wide range of effects on the body and mind, leading to physical, psychological, and emotional changes that can be both immediate and long-lasting. Understanding the different types of drugs and their effects is essential for preventing and treating addiction. In this chapter, we will explore some of the most common types of drugs and their impact on the body and mind.

Stimulants

Stimulants are a class of drugs that increase the activity of the central nervous system, leading to feelings of alertness, energy, and euphoria. Common stimulants include caffeine, nicotine, amphetamines, and cocaine. While these drugs can provide short-term benefits such as increased focus and productivity, they can also have a range of negative effects on the body and mind.

<u>Caffeine</u>: Caffeine is a widely consumed stimulant that is found in coffee, tea, chocolate, and other

products. It works by blocking the activity of adenosine, a neurotransmitter that is responsible for promoting sleep and suppressing arousal. While moderate caffeine intake is generally considered safe, excessive consumption can lead to a range of negative effects, including jitteriness, anxiety, insomnia, and rapid heartbeat.

Nicotine: Nicotine is a highly addictive stimulant that is found in tobacco products. It works by binding to nicotine receptors in the brain, leading to the release of dopamine and other neurotransmitters. While nicotine can provide feelings of relaxation and pleasure, it is also associated with a range of negative health effects, including increased risk of cancer, heart disease, and stroke.

Amphetamines: Amphetamines are a class of synthetic stimulants that are often used to treat attention deficit hyperactivity disorder (ADHD), narcolepsy, and other conditions. They work by increasing the activity of dopamine and other neurotransmitters in the brain, leading to feelings of euphoria, increased alertness, and decreased appetite. However, long-term use of amphetamines can lead to a range of negative effects, including addiction, heart disease, and psychosis.

Cocaine: Cocaine is a highly addictive stimulant that is derived from the coca plant. It works by blocking the reuptake of dopamine and other neurotransmitters, leading to increased levels of these chemicals in the brain. This can result in feelings of pleasure, increased energy, and heightened arousal. However, cocaine use can also lead to a range of negative effects, including addiction, heart disease, and stroke.

Depressants

Depressants are a class of drugs that slow down the activity of the central nervous system, leading to feelings of relaxation, sedation, and decreased anxiety. Common depressants include alcohol, benzodiazepines, and barbiturates. While these drugs can have short-term benefits such as reducing anxiety and promoting sleep, they can also have a range of negative effects on the body and mind.

Alcohol: Alcohol is a widely consumed depressant that is found in beer, wine, and liquor. It works by increasing the activity of the neurotransmitter GABA, leading to feelings of relaxation and sedation. While moderate alcohol consumption is generally considered safe, excessive drinking can lead to a range of negative effects, including liver disease, cancer, and mental health issues.

Benzodiazepines: Benzodiazepines are a class of prescription drugs that are often used to treat anxiety, insomnia, and other conditions. They work by enhancing the activity of GABA in the brain, leading to feelings of relaxation and sedation. However, long-term use of benzodiazepines can lead to a range of negative effects, including addiction, memory problems, depression, and increased risk of falls.

Barbiturates: Barbiturates are a class of sedative-hypnotic drugs that were commonly used to treat anxiety, insomnia, and seizures before the advent of benzodiazepines. They work by depressing the activity of the central nervous system, leading to feelings of relaxation, sedation, and decreased anxiety. However, barbiturates can also be highly addictive and can lead to a range of negative effects, including addiction, depression, memory problems, and overdose.

Opioids

Opioids are a class of drugs that are derived from the opium poppy plant or synthesized in a laboratory. They work by binding to opioid receptors in the brain, leading to feelings of pain relief, euphoria, and sedation. Common opioids include heroin, morphine, oxycodone, and fentanyl. While these drugs can provide short-term pain relief, they can also have a range of negative effects on the body and mind.

Heroin: Heroin is a highly addictive opioid that is typically injected, snorted, or smoked. It works by rapidly crossing the blood-brain barrier and binding to opioid receptors in the brain, leading to feelings of intense pleasure and euphoria. However, heroin use can also lead to a range of negative effects, including addiction, overdose, and increased risk of infectious diseases such as HIV and hepatitis.

<u>Morphine</u>: Morphine is a prescription opioid that is often used to treat severe pain. It works by binding to opioid receptors in the brain and spinal cord, leading to feelings of pain relief and sedation. However, long-term use of morphine can lead to a range of negative effects, including addiction, constipation, and respiratory depression.

<u>Oxycodone</u>: Oxycodone is a prescription opioid that is often used to treat moderate to severe pain. It works by binding to opioid receptors in the brain and spinal cord, leading to feelings of pain relief and euphoria. However, long-term use of oxycodone can lead to a range of negative effects, including addiction, constipation, and respiratory depression.

<u>Fentanyl</u>: Fentanyl is a powerful synthetic opioid that is often used to treat severe pain. It works by binding to opioid receptors in the brain and spinal cord, leading to feelings of pain relief and sedation. However, fentanyl is also associated with a high risk of overdose, as it is many times more potent than other opioids and can quickly lead to respiratory depression and death.

Hallucinogens

Hallucinogens are a class of drugs that can alter perception, thought, and mood. Common hallucinogens include LSD, psilocybin (found in magic mushrooms), and mescaline (found in peyote cactus). While these drugs can provide intense and unique experiences, they can also have a range of negative effects on the body and mind.

LSD: LSD is a powerful hallucinogenic drug that can cause profound changes in perception, thought, and mood. It works by binding to serotonin receptors in the brain, leading to altered sensory experiences and feelings of unity and interconnectedness. However, LSD use can also lead to a range of negative effects, including flashbacks, psychosis, and anxiety.

Psilocybin: Psilocybin is a naturally occurring hallucinogen found in certain types of mushrooms. It works by binding to serotonin receptors in the brain, leading to altered perception and mood. While psilocybin has been shown to have potential therapeutic uses, it can also lead to a range of negative effects, including anxiety, paranoia, and flashbacks.

Mescaline: Mescaline is a naturally occurring hallucinogen found in the peyote cactus. It works by binding to serotonin receptors in the brain.

The cycle of addiction and its impact on the brain

Addiction is a complex and multifaceted disease that affects millions of people around the world. It is characterized by compulsive drug-seeking and drug-taking behavior despite the negative consequences that result from drug use. While addiction is often thought of as a problem of willpower or moral character, it is actually a disease that has a profound impact on the brain and its functioning. In this chapter, we will explore the cycle of addiction and its impact on the brain.

The Cycle of Addiction

The cycle of addiction is a complex and interrelated set of behaviors and thought patterns that can lead to the development and maintenance of addiction. The cycle typically begins with a trigger or cue that prompts the individual to seek out drugs or alcohol. This trigger can be a wide range of factors, including stress, boredom, social pressure, or exposure to drug-related cues such as drug paraphernalia or drug-using friends.

Once the individual has been triggered, they will typically engage in drug-seeking behavior. This can include actively seeking out drugs or alcohol, contacting drug dealers or other sources, or engaging in other activities that are associated with drug use. Once the individual has obtained drugs or alcohol, they will typically experience a period of euphoria or pleasure. This is due to the release of dopamine, a neurotransmitter that is associated with pleasure and reward.

Over time, the individual will develop a tolerance to the drug or alcohol, meaning that they will need to consume larger and larger amounts in order to achieve the same level of euphoria or pleasure. This can lead to an escalating pattern of drug use, where the individual becomes increasingly dependent on the drug or alcohol in order to function.

As the cycle of addiction progresses, the individual will typically experience a range of negative consequences related to their drug use. This can include physical health problems, social isolation, financial problems, legal problems, and problems with mental health. However, despite these negative consequences, the individual will continue to use drugs or alcohol, often at great cost to themselves and those around them.

The Impact of Addiction on the Brain

Addiction has a profound impact on the brain and its functioning. When an individual uses drugs or alcohol, the substances travel to the brain and interact with the brain's reward system. The reward system is a complex network of neurons and neurotransmitters that are responsible for producing feelings of pleasure and reward.

When an individual uses drugs or alcohol, these substances cause a surge in dopamine release in the brain's reward system. This flood of dopamine can produce intense feelings of pleasure and euphoria, which can reinforce the individual's drug-seeking and drug-taking behavior. Over time, the repeated exposure to drugs or alcohol can lead to changes in the brain's reward system, making it less sensitive to natural rewards such as food, sex, or social interaction. This can lead to a situation where the individual is only able to experience pleasure and reward through drug use.

In addition to changes in the brain's reward system, addiction can also lead to changes in other areas of the brain. For example, long-term drug use can lead to changes in the prefrontal cortex, a region of the brain that is responsible for decision-making, impulse control, and other complex cognitive processes. These changes can make it more difficult for the individual to control their drug use and make healthy decisions.

Furthermore, addiction can also lead to changes in the brain's stress response system. When an individual is exposed to stress, the brain releases a cascade of hormones and neurotransmitters that are designed to help the individual cope with the stressor. However, in individuals with addiction, these stress response systems can become dysregulated, leading to increased stress reactivity and a greater risk of relapse.

The role of genetics, environment, and personal factors in addiction

Addiction is a complex disease that is influenced by a wide range of factors, including genetics, environment, and personal factors. In this chapter, we will explore the role that these factors play in the development and maintenance of addiction.

Genetics and Addiction

There is growing evidence to suggest that genetics play a significant role in addiction. Studies of twins and families have shown that there is a heritable component to addiction, meaning that individuals with a family history of addiction are more likely to develop addiction themselves. This heritability is thought to be due to a combination of genetic and environmental factors, with genetic factors accounting for roughly 40-60% of the risk of addiction.

Researchers have identified a number of genes that are associated with an increased risk of addiction. These genes are involved in a wide range of processes, including the regulation of dopamine signaling, the stress response system, and the immune system. However, it is important to note that genetics alone do not determine whether an individual will develop addiction. Environmental factors also play a significant role.

Environment and Addiction

The environment in which an individual lives, works, and socializes can have a significant impact on their risk of developing addiction. Environmental factors that have been shown to increase the risk of addiction include:

- _Exposure to drugs and drug-using peers_: Individuals who are exposed to drugs and drug-using peers are more likely to develop addiction. This is thought to be due to social and environmental factors, as well as genetic factors.

- Stressful life events: Stressful life events, such as trauma, abuse, or the loss of a loved one, can increase the risk of addiction. This is thought to be due to the impact of stress on the brain's reward and stress response systems.

- Availability of drugs: The availability of drugs is a significant factor in the development of addiction. Individuals who live in areas with high rates of drug use and drug availability are more likely to develop addiction.

- <u>Socioeconomic factors:</u> Individuals from lower socioeconomic backgrounds are at increased risk of addiction. This is thought to be due to a range of factors, including increased exposure to stress, reduced access to resources and support, and increased exposure to drugs and drug-using peers.

Personal Factors and Addiction

Personal factors, such as mental health, personality traits, and coping skills, can also play a significant role in the development and maintenance of addiction. Some personal factors that have been shown to increase the risk of addiction include:

- <u>Mental health disorders</u>: Individuals with mental health disorders, such as depression, anxiety, or bipolar disorder, are at increased risk of addiction. This is thought to be due to the impact of these disorders on the brain's reward and stress response systems.

- <u>Impulsivity and sensation-seeking</u>: Individuals who are impulsive and seek out intense sensations are at increased risk of addiction. This is thought to be due to the impact of these traits on the brain's reward and decision-making systems.

- <u>Poor coping skills:</u> Individuals who have poor coping skills, such as difficulty managing stress or regulating their emotions, are at increased risk of addiction. This is thought to be due to the role of drugs in providing temporary relief from stress and negative emotions.

Conclusion

In conclusion, addiction is a complex disease that is influenced by a wide range of factors, including genetics, environment, and personal factors. While genetics play a significant role in addiction, environmental and personal factors also play a crucial role in the development and maintenance of addiction. Understanding the role that these factors play in addiction can help individuals and their loved ones to take steps to reduce their risk of developing addiction, as well as to seek out effective treatment if addiction does develop.

Chapter 2

Seeking Treatment

In this chapter, we will explore the various options available for seeking addiction treatment, as well as the factors that can impact the success of treatment.

The Importance of Seeking Treatment

Seeking treatment for addiction is a critical step in the recovery process. Not only can treatment help individuals overcome their addiction and achieve lasting recovery, but it can also help to address any underlying mental health issues or trauma that may be contributing to their addiction. By seeking treatment, individuals can learn effective coping skills, develop a strong support network, and begin to rebuild their lives.

<u>Types of Addiction Treatment</u>

There are a variety of evidence-based treatments available for addiction, including:

- **Behavioral therapies:** Behavioral therapies, such as cognitive-behavioral therapy (CBT) and contingency management, are designed to help individuals identify and change the thoughts, feelings, and behaviors that contribute to their addiction.

- **Medication-assisted treatment (MAT):** MAT involves the use of medications, such as methadone or buprenorphine, in combination with behavioral therapies to treat addiction to opioids and alcohol.

- **Residential treatment:** Residential treatment programs provide individuals with a supportive and structured environment in which to recover from addiction. These programs typically last for several weeks or months and provide a range of therapies and support services.

- **Outpatient treatment:** Outpatient treatment programs allow individuals to receive treatment while still living at home and attending work or school. These programs typically involve regular therapy sessions and support group meetings.

- **Self-help groups**: Self-help groups, such as Alcoholics Anonymous (AA) and Narcotics Anonymous (NA), provide individuals with a supportive community of peers who are also in recovery from addiction.

Factors That Impact Treatment Success

While seeking treatment for addiction is an important step in the recovery process, it is important to recognize that not all treatment programs are equally effective. There are a variety of factors that can impact the success of addiction treatment, including:

- **Treatment setting**: The setting in which treatment is received can have a significant impact on treatment success. Residential treatment programs, for example, may be more effective for individuals who require a high level of structure and support.

- **Treatment duration:** The length of time that an individual remains in treatment can also impact treatment success. Longer treatment durations are generally associated with better treatment outcomes.

- **Co-occurring mental health issues:** Individuals with co-occurring mental health issues, such as depression or anxiety, may require specialized treatment to effectively address both their addiction and mental health issues.

- **Social support:** The presence of a strong social support network, including friends, family, and support groups, can greatly impact treatment success.

- **Motivation and commitment to recovery:** Finally, an individual's motivation and commitment to recovery are crucial factors in treatment success. Individuals who are highly motivated and committed to their recovery are more likely to succeed in treatment.

Conclusion

Seeking treatment for addiction is a critical step in the recovery process. There are a variety of evidence-based treatments available to help individuals overcome their addiction and achieve lasting recovery. While the success of addiction treatment can be impacted by a variety of factors, including treatment setting, duration, and social support, it is important to recognize that effective treatment is available and that recovery is possible. By seeking treatment and committing to their recovery, individuals can begin to rebuild their lives and achieve lasting sobriety.

Recognizing the signs and symptoms of addiction

We will explore the signs and symptoms of addiction and how to recognize when someone may be struggling with this disease.

Signs and Symptoms of Addiction

1. **Changes in behavior:** One of the most common signs of addiction is changes in behavior. This can include changes in mood, energy level, and sleep patterns. Individuals may become more secretive or isolated, or may exhibit erratic or impulsive behavior.

2. **Loss of interest in activities:** Another common sign of addiction is a loss of interest in activities that were previously enjoyed. This can include hobbies, sports, or social activities.

3. **Physical changes:** Addiction can have physical effects on the body, including changes in appetite, weight, and appearance. Individuals may appear tired or unkempt, or may exhibit symptoms of withdrawal.

4. **Tolerance and withdrawal:** Tolerance and withdrawal are hallmark signs of addiction. Tolerance refers to the need for

increasing amounts of a substance to achieve the same effect, while withdrawal refers to the physical and psychological symptoms that occur when the substance is no longer present.

5. **Continued use despite negative consequences:** Individuals with addiction may continue to use a substance despite negative consequences, such as relationship problems, financial difficulties, or legal issues.

<u>Recognizing Addiction in Others</u>

Recognizing addiction in others can be challenging, as individuals may be hesitant to seek help or may deny that they have a problem. However, there are a few key signs to look for that may indicate that someone is struggling with addiction.

- **Changes in behavior:** As mentioned earlier, changes in behavior can be a key indicator of addiction. If someone you know is exhibiting uncharacteristic behaviors, such as increased secrecy or isolation, it may be a sign that they are struggling with addiction.

- **Loss of interest in activities:** If someone you know has lost interest in activities that they previously enjoyed, it may be a sign of addiction.

- **Changes in appearance:** If someone you know has experienced significant changes in appearance, such as weight loss or a decline in personal hygiene, it may be a sign that they are struggling with addiction.

- **Tolerance and withdrawal:** If someone you know exhibits signs of tolerance or withdrawal, such as needing increasing amounts of a substance to achieve the same effect, or experiencing physical or psychological symptoms when the substance is not present, it may be a sign of addiction.

- **Continued use despite negative consequences:** If someone you know is continuing to use a substance despite negative consequences, it may be a sign that they are struggling with addiction.

Conclusion

In conclusion, recognizing the signs and symptoms of addiction is an important step in helping individuals to seek the support and resources they need to begin the journey towards recovery.

Changes in behavior, loss of interest in activities, physical changes, tolerance and withdrawal, and continued use despite negative consequences are all potential signs of addiction. If you suspect that someone you know may be struggling with addiction, it is important to approach the situation with compassion and empathy, and to encourage them to seek help from a professional or support group. With the right support, individuals with addiction can recover and reclaim their lives.

Approaches to treatment, including medication, therapy, and support groups

we will explore some of the most common approaches to treatment, including medication, therapy, and support groups.

Medication-Assisted Treatment

Medication-assisted treatment (MAT) is an evidence-based approach to treating drug addiction that involves the use of medications to help manage withdrawal symptoms and cravings. MAT is most commonly used for the treatment of opioid addiction, but it can also be effective for other types of addiction.

There are three medications that are commonly used in MAT for opioid addiction: methadone, buprenorphine, and naltrexone. Methadone and buprenorphine are opioid agonists, which means that they work by binding to the same receptors in the brain as opioids. However, because they are longer-acting and have a slower onset of action than most opioids, they can help to prevent withdrawal symptoms and cravings without producing the same euphoric effects.

Naltrexone is an opioid antagonist, which means that it works by blocking the effects of opioids in the brain. Naltrexone does not produce any euphoric effects and is not addictive. It can be used to help prevent relapse in individuals who have already gone through detox and are no longer experiencing withdrawal symptoms.

<u>Behavioral Therapies</u>

Behavioral therapies are a cornerstone of addiction treatment and are often used in combination with medication-assisted treatment. Behavioral therapies aim to help individuals identify the underlying causes of their addiction and develop the skills and strategies needed to manage cravings and avoid relapse.

Cognitive-behavioral therapy (CBT) is one of the most common types of behavioral therapy used in addiction treatment. CBT helps individuals to identify negative thought patterns and develop more positive, constructive ways of thinking. It also helps individuals to develop coping skills that can be used to manage stress and other triggers for drug use.

Motivational interviewing is another approach that is commonly used in addiction treatment. Motivational interviewing aims to help individuals to identify their own reasons for wanting to change and to develop the motivation and confidence needed to make positive changes in their lives.

<u>Support Groups</u>

Support groups are another important component of addiction treatment. Support groups provide individuals with a safe and supportive environment where they can share their experiences, learn from others, and receive encouragement and support.

One of the most well-known support groups for addiction is Alcoholics Anonymous (AA). AA is a self-help group that follows a 12-step program designed to help individuals achieve and maintain sobriety. The group is based on the idea that addiction is a disease that can be managed but not cured, and that recovery is a lifelong process.

Other support groups that may be helpful for individuals with addiction include Narcotics Anonymous (NA), SMART Recovery, and Secular Organizations for Sobriety (SOS).

<u>Conclusion</u>

Drug addiction is a serious and complex disease that requires a multifaceted approach to treatment. Medication-assisted treatment, behavioral therapies, and support groups are all important components of addiction treatment that can be used in combination to help individuals achieve and maintain sobriety. If you or someone you know is struggling with addiction, it is important to seek help from a professional or support group. With the right support and resources, recovery is possible.

Choosing the right treatment program

Choosing the right treatment program for drug addiction can be a daunting task, especially for those who are new to the process. With so many different treatment options available, it can be difficult to know where to start. However, with some research and guidance, individuals and their loved ones can find the treatment program that best suits their needs and helps them achieve lasting recovery. In this chapter, we will explore the key factors to consider when choosing a treatment program for drug addiction.

Levels of Care

One of the first things to consider when choosing a treatment program is the level of care that is needed. The level of care will depend on the severity of the addiction, the presence of co-occurring mental health conditions, and other individual factors. There are several levels of care to choose from, including:

- **Detoxification**: This is the first step in addiction treatment and involves the medical management of withdrawal symptoms. Detoxification is typically a short-term process that lasts anywhere from a few days to a week.

- **Inpatient treatment**: Inpatient treatment involves living at a residential facility while receiving intensive treatment for addiction. Inpatient treatment typically lasts anywhere from 30 to 90 days or more.

- **Partial hospitalization**: Partial hospitalization is a less intensive form of inpatient treatment that involves living at home and attending treatment sessions during the day.

- **Intensive outpatient treatment**: Intensive outpatient treatment involves attending treatment sessions for several hours a day, several days a week.

- **Outpatient treatment**: Outpatient treatment involves attending treatment sessions once or twice a week.

Treatment Approaches

Another factor to consider when choosing a treatment program is the treatment approach that is used. There are several different approaches to addiction treatment, including:

- **Medication-assisted treatment**: Medication-assisted treatment (MAT) involves the use of medications to help manage withdrawal symptoms and cravings. MAT is most commonly used for the treatment of opioid addiction.

- **Behavioral therapies**: Behavioral therapies are a cornerstone of addiction treatment and aim to help individuals identify the underlying causes of their addiction and develop the skills and strategies needed to manage cravings and avoid relapse.

- **Support groups**: Support groups provide individuals with a safe and supportive environment where they can share their experiences, learn from others, and receive encouragement and support.

- **Alternative therapies:** Alternative therapies, such as yoga, meditation, and acupuncture, can also be helpful for some individuals in addiction treatment.

Credentials and Accreditation

When choosing a treatment program, it is important to consider the credentials and accreditation of the facility and its staff. Look for facilities that are accredited by reputable organizations, such as the Commission on Accreditation of Rehabilitation Facilities (CARF) or the Joint Commission. Additionally, make sure that the facility's staff members are licensed and have experience in treating addiction.

Cost and Insurance

The cost of addiction treatment can vary widely depending on the level of care, location, and type of treatment program. Before choosing a treatment program, it is important to consider the cost and whether insurance will cover some or all of the expenses. Many treatment programs accept insurance, but it is important to verify coverage with the insurance provider beforehand.

Location and Amenities

The location of the treatment facility and the amenities it offers can also be important factors to consider. Some individuals may prefer a treatment program that is close to home, while others may prefer to travel to a different location for treatment. Additionally, the amenities offered at the facility, such as a gym, swimming pool, or outdoor recreation area, can help make the treatment experience more comfortable and enjoyable.

Conclusion

Choosing the right treatment program for drug addiction is an important decision that can impact the success of recovery. When choosing a treatment program, consider the level of care, treatment approaches, credentials and accreditation, cost and insurance, and location and amenities. With the right treatment program and support,

Overcoming barriers to treatment, such as stigma and cost

Overcoming barriers to treatment is essential for individuals seeking help for drug addiction. Barriers to treatment can include stigma, cost, access to care, and fear of judgment or discrimination. These barriers can prevent individuals from getting the help they need and can lead to a worsening of their addiction. In this chapter, we will explore some of the common barriers to treatment for drug addiction and offer strategies for overcoming them.

Stigma

Stigma is a major barrier to treatment for drug addiction. Stigma is a negative attitude or belief about a particular group of people, and it can lead to discrimination, prejudice, and marginalization. Individuals with drug addiction often face stigma, which can make it difficult for them to seek help. Some common forms of stigma associated with drug addiction include:

- Blaming the individual for their addiction

- Seeing drug addiction as a moral failing or weakness

- Believing that individuals with drug addiction are dangerous or unpredictable

- Judging individuals with drug addiction for their behavior or lifestyle

To overcome stigma, it is important to educate yourself and others about drug addiction and its causes. Recognize that drug addiction is a disease that affects the brain and the body, and that individuals with drug addiction need treatment and support to recover. You can also challenge stigma by speaking out against it and advocating for policies and programs that support individuals with drug addiction.

Cost

Cost is another common barrier to treatment for drug addiction. Treatment can be expensive, and many individuals with drug addiction may not have the financial resources to pay for it. The cost of treatment can include the cost of medication, therapy, and other support services. Some strategies for overcoming the cost barrier to treatment include:

- Seeking out low-cost or free treatment programs: There are many treatment programs available that offer low-cost or free services for individuals with drug addiction. These programs may be supported by government or community organizations, and can be a great option for individuals who cannot afford traditional treatment programs.

- Looking into insurance coverage: Many insurance providers cover some or all of the cost of addiction treatment. Check with your insurance provider to see what services are covered and what your out-of-pocket costs will be.

- Finding other sources of financial support: There are many organizations that offer financial assistance to individuals with drug addiction who need treatment. These organizations may provide grants, loans, or other types of financial support to help cover the cost of treatment.

Access to Care

Access to care is another barrier to treatment for drug addiction. Some individuals may live in areas where there are few treatment options available, while others may face long wait times for treatment services. Some strategies for overcoming the access to care barrier to treatment include:

- Seeking out telemedicine or online treatment options: Telemedicine and online treatment options can be a great option for individuals who live in areas where there are few treatment options available. These services allow individuals to receive treatment from a distance, which can be especially helpful for individuals who live in rural or remote areas.

- Advocating for increased funding for treatment programs: You can advocate for increased funding for treatment programs in your community or state. This can help increase the availability of treatment services and reduce wait times for care.

Fear of Judgment or Discrimination

Finally, fear of judgment or discrimination can be a major barrier to treatment for drug addiction. Some individuals may be afraid to seek help because they fear being judged or discriminated against because of their addiction. Some strategies for overcoming the fear of judgment or discrimination barrier to treatment include:

- *Seeking out support from a trusted friend or family member*: Having the support of a trusted friend or family member can help individuals feel more comfortable seeking treatment. This support can also help individuals feel less isolated and more connected to their community.

- *Finding a treatment program that offers a safe and supportive environment*: Look for a treatment program that offers a safe and supportive.

Chapter 3

Detox and Withdrawal

Detoxification, or detox, is the process of removing drugs or alcohol from the body. It is an essential first step in the recovery process and can be a difficult and uncomfortable experience for individuals who have been using drugs for a prolonged period. In this chapter, we will explore what detox and withdrawal are, and how they are managed during addiction treatment.

What is Detoxification?

Detoxification is the process of eliminating toxic substances, such as drugs or alcohol, from the body. It can be done in a variety of settings, including inpatient and outpatient treatment programs. The primary goal of detox is to help individuals safely and comfortably withdraw from the drugs they have been using, while managing the physical and psychological symptoms of withdrawal.

Withdrawal Symptoms

Withdrawal symptoms can vary depending on the type of drug that was being used, the length and severity of use, and individual factors such as age and overall health. Common symptoms of withdrawal may include:

- Anxiety
- Depression
- Insomnia
- Nausea
- Vomiting
- Sweating
- Muscle aches
- Cravings

In some cases, withdrawal can be life-threatening, especially if an individual has been using high doses of certain drugs, such as benzodiazepines or alcohol. For this reason, it is important for individuals to undergo detoxification under medical supervision.

<u>Detoxification Methods</u>

There are several methods for detoxification, and the most appropriate method will depend on individual needs and circumstances. Some of the most common methods for detoxification include:

1. Medically Assisted Detox

Medically assisted detox is a supervised process that uses medications to help manage the symptoms of withdrawal. This method is commonly used for individuals who have been using drugs for a long time, or who have a history of severe addiction. Medications such as methadone or buprenorphine may be used to help individuals safely withdraw from opioids, while medications such as benzodiazepines may be used to help individuals withdraw from alcohol.

2. Holistic Detox

Holistic detox is a method that takes a whole-person approach to detoxification. It may include the use of natural remedies, such as herbs and supplements, as well as practices such as yoga, meditation, and acupuncture. Holistic detox aims to support the body's natural detoxification processes while also promoting overall health and wellness.

3. Social Detox

Social detox is a method that relies on support from others to manage the symptoms of withdrawal. This may include staying with friends or family members who can provide emotional support, or participating in a residential treatment program that provides 24-hour support and monitoring.

Regardless of the method used, detoxification is only the first step in the recovery process. It is important for individuals to engage in ongoing treatment and support to maintain sobriety and prevent relapse.

The detoxification process and its challenges

The detoxification process can be challenging both physically and emotionally, as individuals experience a range of withdrawal symptoms that can be uncomfortable and even painful.

1. Withdrawal symptoms can vary depending on the type of drug being used, as well as individual factors such as age, overall health, and length and severity of use.
2. Medically assisted detox can help manage the physical symptoms of withdrawal and reduce the risk of complications, but it is not a cure for addiction.
3. Holistic detox can provide additional support for overall health and wellness during the detoxification process.
4. Social detox can provide emotional support and monitoring to help individuals safely and comfortably withdraw from drugs or alcohol.

Some of the challenges of detoxification may include a lack of access to medical or social support, fear of withdrawal symptoms, and uncertainty about the future.

It is important for individuals to engage in ongoing treatment and support after detoxification to prevent relapse and maintain sobriety.

Withdrawal symptoms and how to manage them

Withdrawal symptoms are the physical and psychological effects that occur when someone who is addicted to a drug abruptly stops using it. These symptoms can be intense and often make it difficult for individuals to quit using drugs on their own. However, with the right support and treatment, it is possible to manage withdrawal symptoms and successfully detox from drugs or alcohol.

Withdrawal symptoms can vary depending on the type of drug being used, as well as individual factors such as age, overall health, and length and severity of use. Some common withdrawal symptoms include:

- Nausea and vomiting
- Diarrhea
- Sweating
- Tremors
- Headaches
- Muscle aches and pains
- Anxiety and irritability
- Depression
- Insomnia
- Cravings

Managing withdrawal symptoms typically involves a combination of medical, emotional, and behavioural approaches. Some of the most effective methods for managing withdrawal symptoms include:

1. *Medical detoxification*: Medical detoxification involves the use of medications to help manage withdrawal symptoms and reduce the risk of complications. Medications may be used to manage symptoms such as nausea, vomiting, and insomnia, and to reduce cravings for drugs. Medical detoxification is typically done in a supervised setting such as a hospital or addiction treatment center.

2. *Nutritional support:* Good nutrition is essential during the detoxification process. Individuals should eat a balanced diet that includes plenty of fruits, vegetables, whole grains, and lean protein. Some people may also benefit from nutritional supplements, such as vitamins and minerals.

3. *Holistic therapies*: Holistic therapies such as acupuncture, massage, and meditation can be helpful in managing withdrawal symptoms. These therapies can help reduce anxiety, alleviate muscle tension, and promote relaxation.

4. *Behavioral therapies:* Behavioral therapies such as cognitive-behavioral therapy (CBT) and motivational interviewing (MI) can be helpful in managing withdrawal symptoms. These therapies can help individuals learn coping skills, manage triggers for drug use, and build a support network to help maintain sobriety.

5. *Support groups:* Support groups such as Alcoholics Anonymous (AA) and Narcotics Anonymous (NA) can be an invaluable source of support during the detoxification process. These groups provide a safe and supportive environment for individuals to share their experiences and connect with others who are going through similar struggles.

It is important to remember that everyone's experience with withdrawal is different. Some people may experience more severe symptoms than others, and some people may find certain treatments more effective than others. It is important to work with a medical professional to develop a personalized treatment plan that addresses your unique needs and goals.

In addition to the above approaches, there are some general tips that can help manage withdrawal symptoms, such as:

- Staying hydrated: Drinking plenty of water and other fluids can help flush toxins out of the body and reduce nausea and headaches.

- Getting plenty of rest: Resting and sleeping can help the body heal and restore its natural balance.

- Engaging in physical activity: Exercise can help reduce anxiety, promote relaxation, and improve mood.

- Avoiding triggers: Triggers such as people, places, or things associated with drug use can increase the risk of relapse. Avoiding these triggers can help reduce the risk of relapse and maintain sobriety.

In conclusion, managing withdrawal symptoms is a crucial part of the detoxification process. With the right support and treatment, it is possible to successfully detox from drugs or alcohol and begin the journey to recovery. It is important to work with a medical professional to develop a personalized treatment plan that addresses your unique needs and goals, and to engage in ongoing treatment and support to maintain sobriety.

Medical supervision and support during detox

Medical supervision and support during detox is crucial for individuals who are seeking to overcome drug addiction. The process of detox can be challenging, and there are various risks involved. It is essential that individuals seeking detox do so under the care of a medical professional to ensure their safety and well-being.

Medical supervision during detox involves having medical professionals available to monitor the patient's vital signs and address any medical concerns that may arise during the detox process. Depending on the type of drug and the severity of the addiction, medical supervision may involve round-the-clock care, medication, and other treatments to manage withdrawal symptoms and minimize discomfort.

One of the main benefits of medical supervision during detox is the ability to manage potentially dangerous withdrawal symptoms. Withdrawal symptoms can range from mild to severe and can include physical symptoms such as nausea, vomiting, and tremors, as well as psychological symptoms such as anxiety, depression, and irritability. In severe cases, withdrawal symptoms can even be life-threatening.

Medical professionals can help manage withdrawal symptoms by providing medications to ease discomfort and prevent complications. For example, medications may be prescribed to manage nausea, reduce anxiety, and prevent seizures. In some cases, medications may be used to help patients gradually wean off addictive drugs and minimize the severity of withdrawal symptoms.

In addition to managing withdrawal symptoms, medical professionals can also provide emotional support and counseling to help patients cope with the challenges of detox. This may involve individual or group therapy, as well as support from trained

Relapse prevention strategies during detox and beyond

While detox is an important first step in overcoming drug addiction, it is only the beginning of a long and challenging journey. Even after detox, individuals in recovery are at risk of relapse, which can set back their progress and undermine their efforts to overcome addiction. That is why it is essential to have effective relapse prevention strategies in place during detox and beyond.

One of the most effective ways to prevent relapse during detox is to remove triggers and temptations from the patient's environment. This may involve moving the patient to a new location, such as a residential treatment facility, where they can receive round-the-clock care and support. It may also involve limiting access to drugs and alcohol and avoiding situations or people that may trigger cravings or temptations.

In addition to environmental factors, there are also psychological and emotional triggers that can contribute to relapse. These may include stress, anxiety, depression, or feelings of isolation or loneliness. To prevent relapse, it is important to address these underlying issues and provide patients with the tools and resources they need to manage them effectively.

Cognitive-behavioral therapy (CBT) is one approach that has been shown to be effective in helping individuals in recovery learn to identify and manage triggers and cravings. Through CBT, patients learn coping strategies to deal with stressful situations, manage negative emotions, and avoid relapse.

Another effective strategy for preventing relapse is to engage in ongoing support and therapy, such as group therapy, 12-step programs, or individual counseling. These programs provide patients with ongoing support and encouragement, helping them to stay on track with their recovery and avoid relapse.

Other strategies for preventing relapse may include developing healthy habits and routines, such as exercise, healthy eating, and mindfulness practices. These activities can help reduce stress, improve mood, and promote overall well-being, all of which can help reduce the risk of relapse.

Finally, it is important to have a plan in place for dealing with potential relapses. While relapse is not uncommon in recovery, it is important to have a plan in place for how to respond to a relapse, including seeking immediate help from medical professionals, therapists, and support groups.

Overall, relapse prevention is an essential component of the recovery process, and individuals in recovery must be proactive in developing and implementing effective strategies for preventing relapse during detox and beyond.

Chapter 4

Therapy and Counseling

Therapy and counseling are important components of the recovery process for individuals struggling with addiction. Therapy and counseling can help individuals to identify and address the underlying issues that contribute to their addiction, such as trauma, mental health issues, or relationship problems.

One of the most effective types of therapy for addiction is **cognitive-behavioral therapy** (CBT). CBT is a form of therapy that focuses on identifying and changing negative thought patterns and behaviors that contribute to addiction. CBT is often used to help individuals in recovery to identify and manage triggers and cravings, develop coping strategies for dealing with stress and negative emotions, and develop a sense of self-efficacy and self-control.

Another type of therapy that can be effective for addiction is **dialectical behavior therapy** (DBT). DBT is a form of therapy that focuses on developing mindfulness, emotion regulation, interpersonal effectiveness, and distress tolerance skills. DBT can be particularly helpful for individuals struggling with addiction and co-occurring mental health issues, such as borderline personality disorder.

Family therapy can also be an effective approach for addiction treatment, particularly for individuals with strong family ties. Family therapy can help individuals in recovery to repair and strengthen relationships with family members, develop better communication and problem-solving skills, and create a support network for recovery.

In addition to therapy, support groups such as 12-step programs can be an effective form of counseling for addiction. 12-step programs provide a supportive and non-judgmental environment for individuals in recovery, where they can share their experiences, receive support, and connect with others who are facing similar challenges.

Another effective approach to counseling for addiction is motivational interviewing (MI). MI is a form of counseling that focuses on helping individuals in recovery to identify and build their own motivation and commitment to change. MI is often used in conjunction with other forms of therapy, such as CBT or DBT, to help individuals in recovery to stay motivated and engaged in their treatment.

Ultimately, the most effective approach to therapy and counseling for addiction will depend on the individual's unique needs and circumstances. It is important for individuals in recovery to work closely with their healthcare providers and therapists to develop a personalized treatment plan that is tailored to their specific needs and goals.

Different types of therapy for addiction treatment, including behavioral therapy, cognitive-behavioral therapy (CBT), and dialectical behavior therapy (DBT)

Addiction is a complex disorder that requires a multifaceted treatment approach. There are many different types of therapy that can be effective in helping individuals overcome addiction and achieve long-term recovery. Here are a few of the most common types of therapy used in addiction treatment:

Behavioral Therapy: Behavioral therapy is a type of therapy that focuses on changing behaviors that are associated with addiction. This type of therapy helps individuals identify and change negative patterns of behavior that contribute to addiction, such as substance use or compulsive behaviors. Behavioral therapy can help individuals develop new coping skills, improve communication, and learn new ways to manage stress and triggers.

- **Cognitive-Behavioral Therapy (CBT):** Cognitive-behavioral therapy (CBT) is a type of therapy that helps individuals identify and change negative thought patterns that contribute to addiction. CBT is based on the idea that negative thoughts and beliefs can lead to negative behaviors, and that changing these thoughts and beliefs can lead to positive changes in behavior. CBT can help individuals identify and manage triggers and cravings, develop coping strategies, and build self-esteem and self-control.

- **Dialectical Behavior Therapy (DBT):** Dialectical behavior therapy (DBT) is a type of therapy that focuses on helping individuals develop skills for managing intense emotions and improving relationships with others. DBT can be particularly helpful for individuals struggling with addiction and co-occurring mental health issues, such as borderline personality disorder. DBT can help individuals develop mindfulness, emotion regulation, interpersonal effectiveness, and distress tolerance skills.

- **Group Therapy**: Group therapy is a type of therapy that involves individuals working together in a group setting. Group therapy can provide a supportive environment where individuals can share their experiences, receive feedback, and build relationships with others who are facing similar challenges. Group therapy can help individuals develop a sense of community and support, which can be an important component of recovery.

- **Family Therapy:** Family therapy is a type of therapy that involves the individual in recovery and their family members. Family therapy can help individuals repair and strengthen relationships with family members, develop better communication and problem-solving skills, and create a support network for recovery. Family therapy can be particularly effective for individuals with strong family ties.

- **Motivational Interviewing (MI):** Motivational interviewing (MI) is a type of therapy that focuses on helping individuals in recovery identify and build their own motivation and commitment to change. MI can be particularly helpful for individuals who are ambivalent about making changes or who are resistant to treatment. MI can help individuals stay motivated and engaged in their treatment.

Ultimately, the most effective type of therapy for addiction treatment will depend on the individual's unique needs and circumstances. It is important for individuals in recovery to work closely with their healthcare providers and therapists to develop a personalized treatment plan that is tailored to their specific needs and goals.

The role of counseling in addiction recovery

Counseling is a crucial aspect of addiction recovery. It can help individuals identify the underlying issues that contributed to their addiction and develop coping mechanisms to prevent relapse. Counseling is often provided as part of a comprehensive treatment program that includes medical and therapeutic interventions.

Counseling can take different forms, depending on the individual's needs and preferences. One of the most common types of counseling for addiction is individual counseling, which involves working one-on-one with a licensed therapist or counselor. In this type of counseling, the therapist helps the individual identify the root causes of their addiction and develop a plan to overcome it.

Another type of counseling is group therapy, which involves working with a group of people who are all dealing with addiction. In group therapy, individuals can share their experiences and provide support to one another. Group therapy can also help individuals learn from one another's successes and challenges.

Family therapy is another type of counseling that is often used in addiction treatment. In family therapy, the individual and their family members work together with a therapist to address issues that may have contributed to the addiction. Family therapy can help improve communication and relationships, which can be key to a successful recovery.

Counseling can be provided in various settings, such as inpatient and outpatient treatment centers, as well as private practices. It is important to find a therapist or counselor who specializes in addiction treatment and who is a good fit for the individual's needs and personality.

Overall, counseling can play a vital role in addiction recovery by helping individuals understand the underlying issues that led to their addiction, developing coping mechanisms to prevent relapse, and improving relationships with family and friends.

Addressing co-occurring mental health conditions and trauma

Many individuals struggling with addiction also have co-occurring mental health conditions or have experienced trauma in their lives. It is important to address these underlying issues to achieve successful addiction recovery.

Mental health conditions such as anxiety, depression, bipolar disorder, and post-traumatic stress disorder (PTSD) are often linked with addiction. If left untreated, these conditions can make it more difficult for individuals to overcome addiction. Integrated treatment programs that address both addiction and mental health conditions have been shown to be more effective than treatment programs that focus solely on addiction.

Trauma is another issue that can contribute to addiction. Trauma can include experiences such as physical, emotional, or sexual abuse, neglect, violence, or natural disasters. Trauma can cause individuals to turn to drugs or alcohol as a coping mechanism. To address addiction, it is important to address the underlying trauma.

Counseling can be an effective way to address co-occurring mental health conditions and trauma. Therapists who specialize in trauma and addiction can provide evidence-based treatment, such as cognitive processing therapy (CPT) and eye movement desensitization and reprocessing (EMDR), which can help individuals process and overcome trauma.

In addition to counseling, medication-assisted treatment (MAT) can be helpful in treating co-occurring mental health conditions and addiction. MAT involves the use of medications, such as antidepressants or anti-anxiety medications, to address mental health conditions while also treating addiction.

Overall, addressing co-occurring mental health conditions and trauma is a critical component of addiction recovery. By providing comprehensive treatment that addresses both addiction and underlying issues, individuals can achieve long-term recovery and improve their overall quality of life.

Developing coping skills and healthy habits

Developing coping skills and healthy habits is an essential part of addiction recovery. Coping skills can help individuals manage stress and avoid triggers that can lead to relapse, while healthy habits can improve overall physical and mental health.

Some examples of coping skills that can be helpful for addiction recovery include:

<u>Mindfulness</u>: Mindfulness involves being present in the moment and focusing on your thoughts, feelings, and bodily sensations. This can help

individuals become more aware of their triggers and manage stress more effectively.

<u>Exercise</u>: Exercise can help reduce stress, improve mood, and increase overall physical health. It can also help individuals build self-confidence and self-esteem, which can be important in addiction recovery.

<u>Meditation</u>: Meditation can help individuals manage stress, reduce anxiety and depression, and improve overall mental health.

<u>Creative outlets</u>: Engaging in creative activities such as writing, art, or music can help individuals express themselves and manage stress in a healthy way.

<u>Social support</u>: Building a support system of family, friends, and peers who are supportive of addiction recovery can be helpful in managing stress and avoiding triggers.

Healthy habits that can be helpful in addiction recovery include:

<u>Getting enough sleep</u>: Lack of sleep can increase stress and make it more difficult to manage cravings and triggers.

<u>Eating a healthy diet</u>: Eating a healthy diet can improve overall physical and mental health, and

can also help individuals manage cravings and avoid triggers.

<u>Avoiding drugs and alcohol:</u> It is important to avoid drugs and alcohol in order to maintain sobriety and avoid triggers.

<u>Practicing self-care:</u> Practicing self-care activities such as taking a warm bath, getting a massage, or practicing yoga can help individuals manage stress and promote overall physical and mental health.

Staying engaged in positive activities: Staying engaged in positive activities such as hobbies, volunteer work, or education can help individuals stay motivated and maintain a sense of purpose in their recovery.

Overall, developing coping skills and healthy habits is an important part of addiction recovery. By incorporating these strategies into their daily lives, individuals can improve their overall physical and mental health, manage stress and triggers, and maintain long-term sobriety.

Chapter 5

Support Groups and Community Resources

The importance of peer support in addiction recovery

Addiction recovery can be a challenging and isolating journey, which is why peer support is so important. Peer support involves connecting with others who have gone through similar experiences and can provide encouragement, guidance, and empathy. Peer support can come in many forms, including support groups, recovery communities, and sober living homes.

One of the most well-known forms of peer support is 12-step programs, such as Alcoholics Anonymous (AA) and Narcotics Anonymous (NA). These programs provide a supportive environment where individuals can connect with others who are also in recovery, share their experiences, and receive guidance from others who have gone through similar experiences. In addition, these programs provide a structured approach to recovery that can help individuals stay focused on their goals.

In recent years, there has been a growing recognition of the importance of peer support beyond 12-step programs. Recovery communities, such as online forums and social media groups, can provide a sense of community and connection for individuals in recovery. These communities can also provide access to resources and support for individuals who may not have access to traditional support groups.

Sober living homes are another form of peer support that can be helpful for individuals in recovery. Sober living homes provide a structured and supportive environment where individuals can live with others who are also in recovery. This can provide a sense of community and accountability that can be helpful in maintaining sobriety.

One of the key benefits of peer support is that it can help individuals feel less alone in their recovery journey. Connecting with others who have gone through similar experiences can provide a sense of understanding and empathy that can be difficult to find in other settings. In addition, peer support can provide practical guidance and support for navigating the challenges of recovery.

It is important to note that peer support is not a replacement for professional treatment. However, peer support can be a valuable supplement to professional treatment and can provide additional support and guidance for individuals in recovery. By connecting with others who have gone through similar experiences, individuals can build a sense of community and support that can be essential in achieving and maintaining sobriety.

Different types of support groups, including 12-step programs and non-12-step programs

Support groups can be an important aspect of addiction recovery, providing individuals with a community of people who understand the challenges of addiction and can offer guidance, support, and encouragement. There are a variety of different support groups available, each with its own unique approach and focus.

One of the most well-known types of support groups is the 12-step program, which was first developed by Alcoholics Anonymous (AA). 12-step programs are based on the belief that addiction is a disease that requires ongoing treatment and support. These programs involve a series of steps that individuals work through in order to achieve and maintain sobriety. Some of the most well-known 12-step programs include Alcoholics Anonymous (AA) and Narcotics Anonymous (NA).

While 12-step programs can be a helpful form of support for many individuals, they are not the only option available. Non-12-step support groups are becoming increasingly popular, offering a different approach to addiction recovery. These groups may focus on topics such as mindfulness, cognitive-behavioral therapy, or holistic healing. Some of the most well-known non-12-step support groups include SMART Recovery and LifeRing.

SMART Recovery is a non-profit organization that provides support for individuals seeking to overcome addiction and other problematic behaviors. The organization uses a cognitive-behavioral approach, which focuses on identifying and changing negative thought patterns and behaviors. SMART Recovery meetings are led by trained facilitators who provide guidance and support for individuals in recovery.

LifeRing is another non-12-step support group that offers an alternative to traditional 12-step programs. The organization provides support for individuals in recovery through a secular approach that focuses on personal responsibility and self-empowerment. LifeRing meetings are led by trained facilitators who provide a supportive and non-judgmental environment for individuals in recovery.

In addition to 12-step and non-12-step programs, there are a variety of other support groups available for individuals in recovery. These may include groups focused on specific types of addiction, such as gambling addiction or sex addiction, as well as groups for individuals who have experienced trauma or other mental health challenges.

One of the key benefits of support groups is the sense of community and connection they provide. By connecting with others who have gone through similar experiences, individuals can feel less alone in their recovery journey and can receive guidance and support from others who understand the challenges of addiction. Whether an individual chooses a 12-step program or a non-12-step program, the important thing is that they find a support group that feels like a good fit for their needs and that can provide the support and guidance they need to achieve and maintain sobriety.

Finding and connecting with support groups in your community

Finding and connecting with support groups in your community is an essential step in addiction recovery. There are different types of support groups available, both 12-step and non-12-step programs, each with its own unique approach to recovery. These groups can provide a sense of community, support, and encouragement to individuals in recovery, as well as a space to share experiences and learn from others who have gone through similar struggles.

One of the most well-known types of support groups is the 12-step program, which was founded by Alcoholics Anonymous (AA) in 1935. Today, there are many different 12-step programs for different types of addictions, such as Narcotics Anonymous (NA), Cocaine Anonymous (CA), and Gamblers Anonymous (GA), among others. These programs are based on a set of 12 principles and offer a structured approach to recovery, including regular meetings, working through the 12 steps with a sponsor, and developing a spiritual practice.

While 12-step programs have helped many people achieve and maintain sobriety, they are not the only option available. Non-12-step programs offer a different approach to recovery, often focusing on building personal responsibility, self-awareness, and self-empowerment. Some examples of non-12-step programs include SMART Recovery, LifeRing Secular Recovery, and Women for Sobriety. These programs often offer online and in-person meetings, as well as tools and resources for self-help and recovery.

When looking for a support group in your community, it is important to consider what type of group and approach will work best for you. You can start by asking for recommendations from a therapist or counselor, contacting local treatment centers or community organizations, or searching online for local support groups. Many support groups also have websites or social media pages where you can find more information about meeting times, locations, and the group's approach to recovery.

Once you have found a support group that you are interested in, it can be helpful to attend a meeting to get a sense of the group's atmosphere and approach. While it can be intimidating to attend a meeting for the first time, remember that everyone in the room has been where you are and is there to offer support and encouragement. It is also important to remember that finding the right support group may take some trial and error, and it is okay to try different groups until you find one that feels like a good fit.

In addition to support groups, there are also many other ways to connect with others in recovery and build a supportive community. This can include attending sober events, joining a recreational or hobby group, or volunteering for a local organization. The important thing is to find ways to connect with others in a positive and supportive environment, as this can help to reduce feelings of isolation and promote a sense of purpose and fulfillment in recovery.

Overall, finding and connecting with support groups in your community is an essential part of addiction recovery. Whether you choose a 12-step or non-12-step program, the support, encouragement, and sense of community that these groups offer can be a valuable asset in maintaining sobriety and building a fulfilling life in recovery.

Other resources for addiction recovery, such as online forums and helplines

While support groups can be incredibly helpful for those in addiction recovery, it's important to remember that they are not the only resources available. There are a variety of other resources that can provide additional support and guidance for those in need.

One such resource is online forums. Online forums provide a platform for individuals to connect with others who are going through similar experiences. Many of these forums are moderated by professionals and provide a safe and supportive space for people to discuss their struggles and share their stories. In addition, online forums can be accessed at any time, making them a convenient option for those who may not have the time or resources to attend in-person meetings.

Another valuable resource for those in addiction recovery is helplines. Helplines provide a confidential and immediate source of support for those who may be struggling with addiction or in need of assistance. These helplines are staffed by trained professionals who can provide information, guidance, and referrals to treatment resources. In addition, many helplines operate 24/7, making them a great option for those who may be in crisis outside of regular business hours.

When it comes to finding online forums and helplines, there are a variety of resources available. Many organizations and treatment centers offer lists of online forums and helplines on their websites. In addition, a simple online search can yield a variety of results. It's important to carefully evaluate any resources before using them to ensure they are reputable and provide reliable information and support.

In addition to online forums and helplines, there are a variety of other resources available for those in addiction recovery. Many treatment centers offer aftercare programs that provide ongoing support and guidance for individuals who have completed treatment. In addition, there are a variety of educational resources available that can help individuals learn more about addiction and how to manage it.

Overall, it's important to remember that addiction recovery is a journey and there are a variety of resources available to help individuals along the way. Whether it's through support groups, online forums, helplines, or other resources, it's important to seek out the help and guidance that is needed to achieve and maintain recovery.

Chapter 6

Maintaining Recovery

Strategies for maintaining sobriety and preventing relapse

Achieving sobriety is a significant accomplishment for anyone who has struggled with addiction. However, it's important to recognize that recovery is a lifelong journey, and maintaining sobriety requires ongoing effort and dedication. In this chapter, we will explore strategies that can help you stay on track and avoid relapse.

<u>Develop a Strong Support System</u>

Having a strong support system is crucial for maintaining sobriety. This can include friends, family, and peers who are also in recovery. It's essential to surround yourself with people who are supportive, understanding, and non-judgmental. These people can provide encouragement and accountability, which can be incredibly valuable in helping you stay sober.

Continue Therapy and Counseling

Therapy and counseling can be instrumental in maintaining sobriety. Continuing to work with a therapist or counselor can help you process any underlying issues that may have contributed to your addiction. Additionally, it can help you develop coping skills, improve your emotional regulation, and build self-awareness, which are all critical components of a successful recovery.

Identify Triggers and High-Risk Situations

It's essential to identify triggers and high-risk situations that may lead to relapse. This can include anything from stress, anxiety, and depression to specific people, places, and events. Once you identify your triggers, you can work with your therapist or counselor to develop a plan for managing them effectively.

Practice Self-Care

Self-care is an important part of maintaining sobriety. This can include anything from exercise, healthy eating, and meditation to spending time with loved ones and engaging in enjoyable hobbies. Taking care of yourself both physically and mentally can help reduce stress and anxiety, which are common triggers for relapse.

Accountability is critical in maintaining sobriety. This can include attending support group meetings, working with a sponsor, or sharing your recovery journey with a trusted friend or family member. When you are accountable to others, it can help keep you focused on your goals and provide the motivation to stay sober.

Create a Plan for Relapse Prevention

It's essential to have a plan in place for preventing relapse. This can include developing a list of coping strategies, identifying the signs of relapse, and having a plan for what to do if you feel at risk of relapse. Additionally, it's essential to have a support system in place that you can turn to if you need help.

Celebrate Milestones and Progress

Recovery is a challenging journey, and it's essential to celebrate the milestones and progress you make along the way. This can include anything from celebrating your sobriety anniversary to recognizing the positive changes you've made in your life. Celebrating your achievements can help provide motivation and reinforce your commitment to sobriety.

Lifestyle changes to support recovery, including exercise, nutrition, and self-care

Maintaining sobriety and preventing relapse requires a holistic approach that addresses not only the addiction but also the individual's lifestyle and overall health. A healthy lifestyle can support recovery and help prevent relapse. It is important to develop new habits and routines that support sobriety, such as exercise, nutrition, and self-care.

Exercise is an essential part of a healthy lifestyle, and it can also be an effective tool in maintaining sobriety. Exercise can improve mood and reduce stress and anxiety, which are often triggers for substance use. It can also help boost self-esteem and confidence, both of which are crucial in recovery. Exercise does not have to be intense or time-consuming; even short, regular walks can be beneficial. Finding an exercise that is enjoyable and sustainable is key to making it a regular part of a healthy lifestyle.

Nutrition is another essential part of a healthy lifestyle. Substance abuse can often take a toll on an individual's physical health, leading to poor nutrition and overall wellness. A healthy diet can help improve physical and mental health, which can aid in recovery. Eating a balanced diet that includes plenty of fruits and vegetables, whole grains, and lean protein can help provide the necessary nutrients to support physical and mental health.

Self-care is also crucial in maintaining sobriety and preventing relapse. It involves taking care of oneself physically, mentally, and emotionally. This can include practicing relaxation techniques, such as meditation or deep breathing exercises, getting enough sleep, and engaging in activities that bring joy and fulfillment. Self-care is important in reducing stress and managing triggers that can lead to substance use.

It is also important to identify and avoid triggers that may lead to relapse. Triggers can be anything from people, places, or situations that may lead to cravings or a desire to use drugs or alcohol. Developing healthy coping mechanisms to manage triggers, such as practicing mindfulness or reaching out to a support group, can be effective in preventing relapse.

In addition, developing a strong support system can be essential in maintaining sobriety. This can include family, friends, peers in recovery, or a sponsor in a 12-step program. It is important to surround oneself with people who support sobriety and understand the challenges of recovery.

In conclusion, maintaining sobriety and preventing relapse requires a multifaceted approach that addresses all aspects of an individual's health and lifestyle. Incorporating regular exercise, healthy nutrition, self-care, and avoiding triggers can be effective strategies in maintaining sobriety. Additionally, building a strong support system can provide the necessary emotional support to overcome challenges and maintain a successful recovery.

Building a support network and seeking ongoing treatment as needed

Achieving sobriety is a significant accomplishment, but it is only the beginning of a lifelong journey in recovery. Maintaining sobriety and preventing relapse require continued effort, commitment, and support. Building a strong support network and seeking ongoing treatment as needed are essential strategies for sustaining recovery and preventing relapse.

One of the most crucial steps in maintaining sobriety is building a strong support network. Support can come in many forms, including family, friends, peers, sponsors, therapists, and support groups. These individuals and groups can provide a sense of community, encouragement, and accountability, making it easier to stay on track with recovery goals.

Family and friends can offer unconditional love and support, but it is also essential to connect with others who have been through similar experiences. Peer support groups like 12-step programs, SMART Recovery, and Refuge Recovery can provide a sense of belonging, camaraderie, and the opportunity to share experiences, strength, and hope.

A sponsor, typically someone who has already completed the program, can offer guidance and support in navigating the challenges of recovery. A therapist can provide a safe and supportive environment for addressing underlying mental health issues, developing coping skills, and processing difficult emotions.

It is essential to remain connected to these support systems even as recovery progresses. Recovery is not a one-time event, but an ongoing process that requires continued effort and dedication. Continuing to attend support group meetings, participating in therapy, and maintaining contact with sponsors and sober friends can help maintain a sense of accountability and motivation.

In addition to building a strong support network, seeking ongoing treatment as needed can also help prevent relapse. Addiction is a chronic disease that requires ongoing management, just like any other chronic health condition. Ongoing treatment may include continuing therapy or counseling, attending support group meetings, taking medication as prescribed, and seeking out additional treatment as needed.

Regular check-ins with a primary care physician or addiction specialist can help monitor physical health and address any medical issues that may arise. Co-occurring mental health disorders, such as depression or anxiety, may require ongoing medication management and therapy to prevent relapse.

It is essential to recognize that addiction is a chronic disease that requires ongoing attention and management. Maintaining sobriety and preventing relapse requires ongoing commitment, effort, and support. Building a strong support network, seeking ongoing treatment as needed, and remaining connected to recovery resources can help make the journey in recovery a lifelong success.

Conclusion

Healing from drug addiction is a journey that requires commitment, patience, and a willingness to seek help. With the right approach, it is possible to overcome addiction and lead a fulfilling life in recovery. This book has provided a comprehensive guide on understanding addiction, seeking treatment, and maintaining recovery. Remember, you are not alone in your journey towards healing. There are resources and support available to help you every step of the way.

About the author

Steve Davis is an author and addiction recovery specialist who has written a powerful book on overcoming drug addiction. In his book, titled "The Complete Guide to Addiction Recovery: Your Path to Healing, Hope, and Happiness," Davis draws upon his decades of experience in the field of addiction recovery to provide readers with a comprehensive and practical guide to breaking free from the grips of addiction.

One of the key strengths of Davis' book is his ability to explain the science behind addiction in a way that is easy to understand. He explains how drugs and alcohol affect the brain and body, leading to addiction and the difficulties that come with it. Davis also goes into detail about the many different factors that can contribute to addiction, including genetic predisposition, trauma, and environmental factors.

But Davis doesn't just focus on the science of addiction. He also provides readers with a step-by-step plan for overcoming addiction and building a fulfilling life in recovery. He offers guidance on how to detox safely and effectively, and he provides practical advice on how to manage the challenges that often arise during the recovery process.

Throughout the book, Davis emphasizes the importance of a holistic approach to addiction recovery. He encourages readers to not only address their physical dependence on drugs or alcohol, but also to work on their mental and emotional health, as well as their social connections and spiritual well-being. He provides tools and resources for addressing these different aspects of recovery, including mindfulness practices, therapy, support groups, and more.

Perhaps most importantly, Davis offers hope to those who may feel like they are stuck in a cycle of addiction. He shares stories of real people who have successfully overcome addiction and rebuilt their lives, and he encourages readers to believe that they too can do the same. He reminds readers that recovery is not a linear process, and that setbacks are a normal part of the journey.

In conclusion, Steve Davis' book on addiction recovery is an invaluable resource for anyone who is struggling with addiction or who knows someone who is. Davis' comprehensive

approach to recovery, combined with his years
of experience in the field, make this book a
must-read for anyone who is ready to take the
first steps towards a fulfilling life in recovery.

www.ingramcontent.com/pod-product-compliance
Lightning Source LLC
Chambersburg PA
CBHW061323250726
48653CB00037BA/2358